My Diabetic Soup & Stew Cookbook

An Unmissable Collection of Easy, Healthy & Delicious Diabetic Recipes

Valerie Blanchard

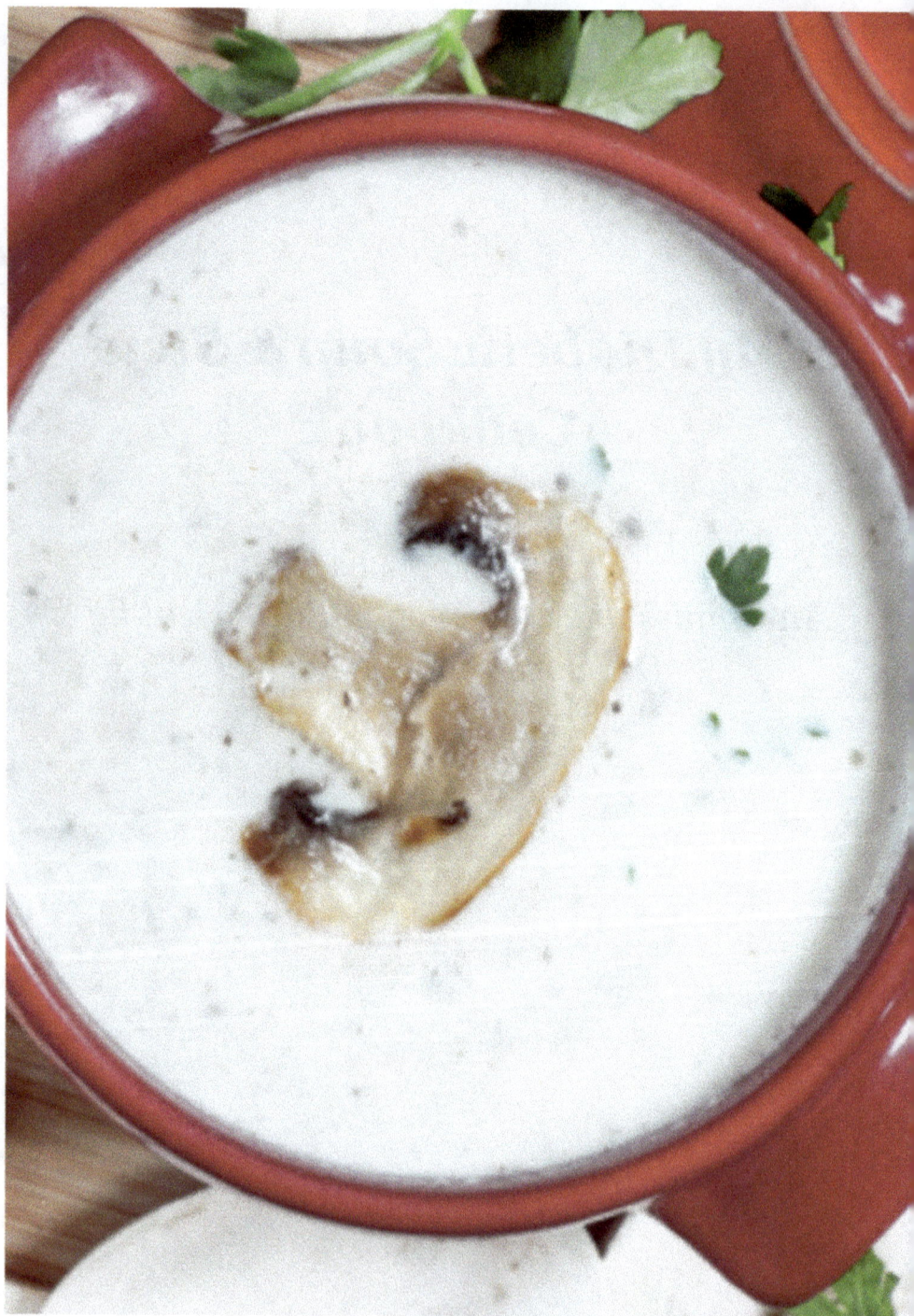

Table of Contents

Pumpkin and White Bean Soup with Sage

Preparation Time: 10 minutes

Cooking Time: 40 minutes

Servings: 3-4

Ingredients:

- 1 ½ pound pumpkin

- ½ pound yams

- ½ pound white beans

- 1 onion

- 2 cloves of garlic

- 1 tbsp. of cold squeezed additional virgin olive oil

- 1 tbsp. of spices (your top picks)

- 1 tbsp. of sage

- 1 ½ quart water (best: antacid water)

- A spot of ocean salt and pepper

Directions:

1. Cut the pumpkin and potatoes in shapes, cut the onion and cut the garlic, the spices and the sage in fine pieces.

2. Sauté the onion and also the garlic in olive oil for around two or three minutes.

3. Include the potatoes, pumpkin, spices and sage and fry for an additional 5 minutes.

4. At that point include the water and cook for around 30 minutes (spread the pot with a top) until vegetables are delicate.

5. At long last include the beans and some salt and pepper. Cook for an additional 5 minutes and serve right away. Prepared!! Appreciate this antacid soup. Alkalizing tasty!

Nutrition: Calories: 78; Carbohydrates: 12g

Alkaline Carrot Soup with Millet

Preparation Time: 7 minutes

Cooking Time: 40 minutes

Servings: 3-4

Ingredients:

- 2 cups cauliflower pieces

- 1 cup potatoes, cubed

- 2 cups vegetables stock (without yeast)

- 3 tbsp. Swiss Emmenthal cheddar, cubed

- 2 tbsp. new chives

- 1 tbsp. pumpkin seeds

1 touch of nutmeg and cayenne pepper

Directions:

1. Cook cauliflower and potato in vegetable stock until delicate and Blend with a blender.

2. Season the soup with nutmeg and cayenne, and possibly somewhat salt and pepper.

3. Include Emmenthal cheddar and chives and mix a couple of moments until the soup is smooth and prepared to serve. Can enhance with pumpkin seeds.

Nutrition: Calories: 65; Carbohydrates: 15g; Fat: 1g; Protein: 2g

Alkaline Pumpkin Tomato Soup

Preparation Time: 15 minutes

Cooking Time: 30 minutes

Servings: 3-4

Ingredients:

- 1 quart of water (if accessible: soluble water)

- 400g new tomatoes, stripped and diced

- 1 medium-sized sweet pumpkin

- 5 yellow onions

- 1 tbsp. Cold squeezed additional virgin olive oil

- 2 tsp. ocean salt or natural salt

- Touch of Cayenne pepper

- Your preferred spices (discretionary)

- Bunch of new parsley

Directions:

1. Cut onions in little pieces and sauté with some oil in a significant pot.

2. Cut the pumpkin down the middle, at that point remove the stem and scoop out the seeds.

3. At long last scoop out the fragile living creature and put it in the pot.

4. Include likewise the tomatoes and the water and cook for around 20 minutes.

5. At that point empty the soup into a food processor and blend well for a couple of moments. Sprinkle with salt pepper and other spices.

6. Fill bowls and trimming with new parsley. Make the most of your alkalizing soup!

Nutrition: Calories: 78; Carbohydrates: 20; Fat: 0.5g; Protein: 1.5g

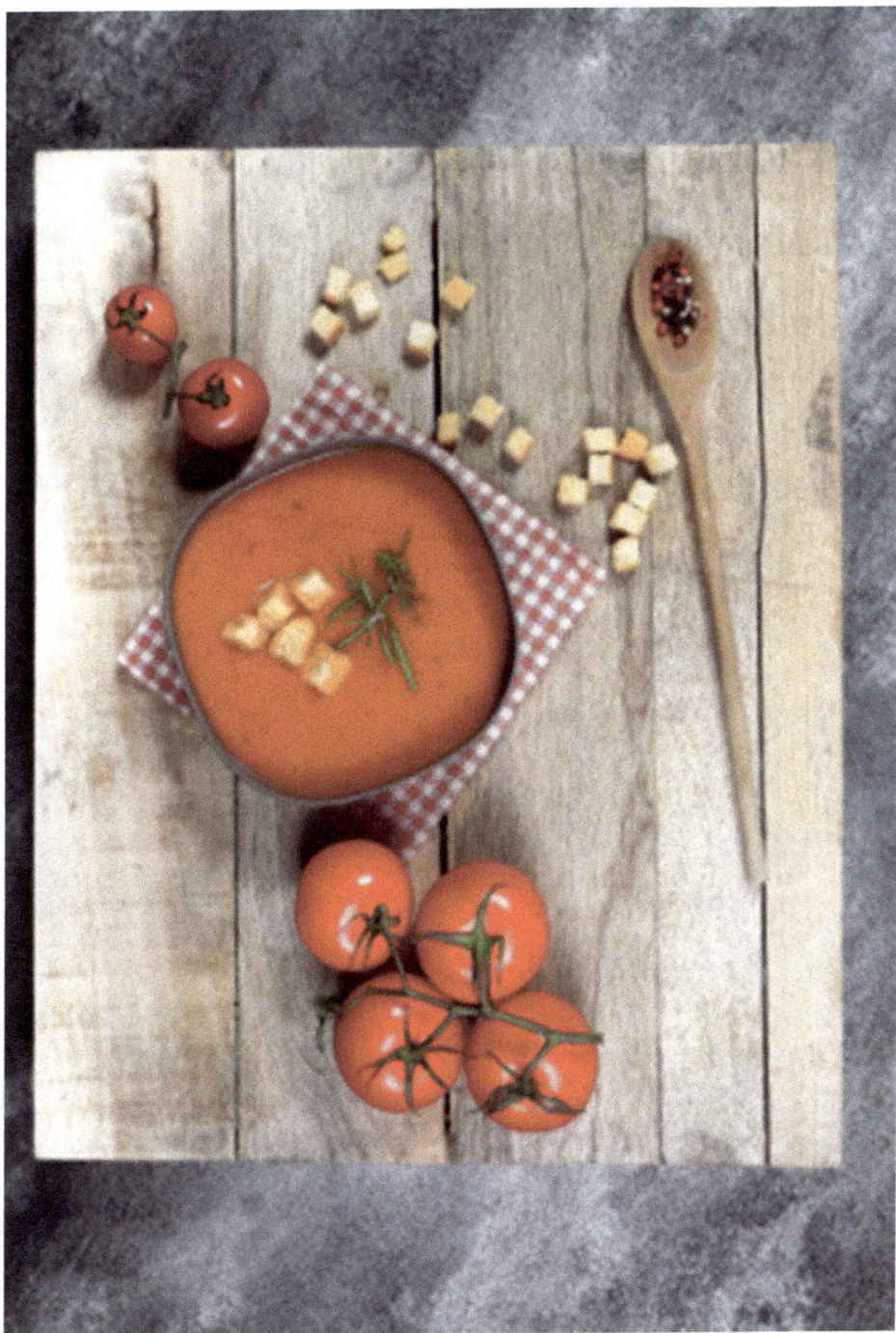

Alkaline Pumpkin Coconut Soup

__Preparation Time:__ 10 minutes

__Cooking Time__: 15 minutes

__Servings:__ 3-4

Ingredients:

- 2lb pumpkin

- 6 cups water (best: soluble water delivered with a water ionizer)

- 1 cup low fat coconut milk

- 5 ounces potatoes

- 2 major onions

- 3 ounces leek

- 1 bunch of new parsley

- 1 touch of nutmeg

- 1 touch of cayenne pepper

- 1 tsp. ocean salt or natural salt

- 4 tbsp. cold squeezed additional virgin olive oil

Directions:

1. As a matter of first significance: cut the onions, the pumpkin, and the potatoes just as the hole into little pieces.

2. At that point, heat the olive oil in a significant pot and sauté the onions for a couple of moments.

3. At that point include the water and heat up the pumpkin, potatoes and the leek until delicate.

4. Include the coconut milk.

5. Presently utilize a hand blender and puree for around 1 moment. The soup should turn out to be extremely velvety.

6. Season with salt, pepper and nutmeg lastly include the parsley. 7. Appreciate this alkalizing pumpkin soup hot or cold!

Nutrition: Calories: 88; Carbohydrates: 23g; Fat: 2.5 g;
Protein: 1.8g

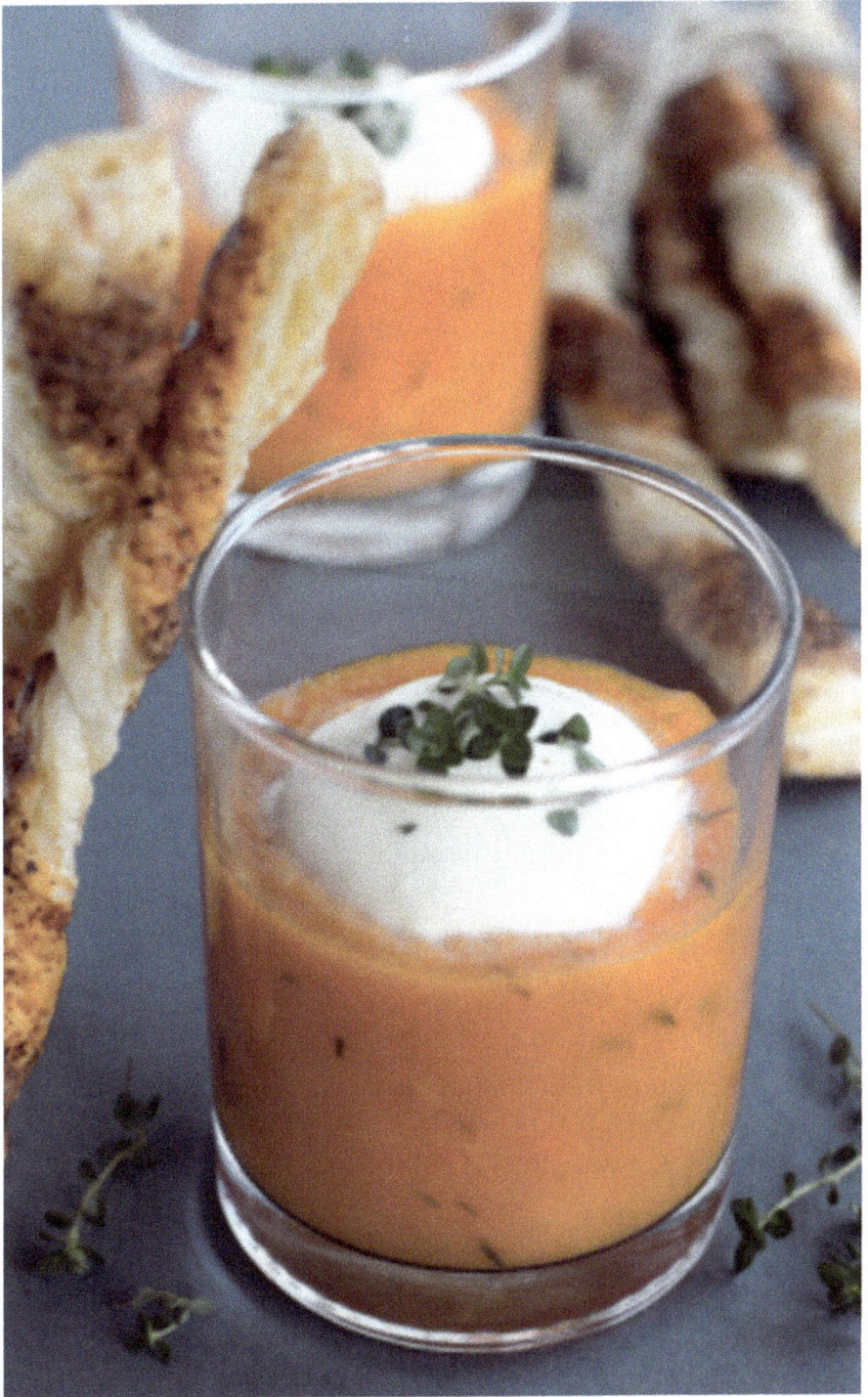

Cold Cauliflower-Coconut Soup

Preparation Time: 7 minutes

Cooking Time: 20 minutes

Servings: 3-4

Ingredients:

- 1 pound (450g) new cauliflower

- 1 ¼ cup (300ml) unsweetened coconut milk

- 1 cup water (best: antacid water)

- 2 tbsp. new lime juice

- 1/3 cup cold squeezed additional virgin olive oil

- 1 cup new coriander leaves, slashed

- Spot of salt and cayenne pepper

- 1 bunch of unsweetened coconut chips

Directions:

1. Steam cauliflower for around 10 minutes.

2. At that point, set up the cauliflower with coconut milk and water in a food processor and procedure until extremely smooth.

3. Include new lime squeeze, salt and pepper, a large portion of the cleaved coriander and the oil and blend for an additional couple of moments.

4. Pour in soup bowls and embellishment with coriander and coconut chips. Appreciate!

Nutrition: Calories: 65; Carbohydrates: 11g; Fat: 0.3g; Protein: 1.5g

Raw Avocado-Broccoli Soup with Cashew Nuts

Preparation Time: 10 minutes

Cooking Time: 30 minutes

Servings: 1-2

Ingredients:

- ½ cup water (if available: alkaline water)

- ½ avocado

- 1 cup chopped broccoli

- ½ cup cashew nuts

- ½ cup alfalfa sprouts

- 1 clove of garlic

- 1 tbsp. cold pressed extra virgin olive oil

- 1 pinch of sea salt and pepper

- Some parsley to garnish

Directions:

1. Put the cashew nuts in a blender or food processor, include some water and puree for a couple of moments.

2. Include the various fixings (with the exception of the avocado) individually and puree each an ideal opportunity for a couple of moments.

3. Dispense the soup in a container and warm it up to the normal room temperature. Enhance with salt and pepper. In the interim dice the avocado and slash the parsley.

4. Dispense the soup in a container or plate; include the avocado dices and embellishment with parsley.

5. That's it! Enjoy this excellent healthy soup!

Nutrition: Calories: 48; Carbohydrates: 18g; Fat: 3g; Protein: 1.4g

White Bean Soup

__Preparation Time:__ 10 minutes

__Cooking Time__: 40 minutes

Servings: 6

Ingredients:

- 2 cups white beans, rinsed

- ¼ tsp. cayenne pepper

- 1 tsp. dried oregano

- ½ tsp. fresh rosemary, chopped

- 3 cups filtered alkaline water

- 3 cups unsweetened almond milk

- 3 garlic cloves, minced

- 2 celery stalks, diced

- 1 onion, chopped

- 1 tbsp. olive oil

- ½ tsp. sea salt

Directions:

1. Add oil into the instant pot and set the pot on sauté mode.

2. Add carrots, celery, and onion in oil and sauté until softened, about 5 minutes.

3. Add garlic and sauté for a minute.

4. Add beans, seasonings, water, and almond milk and stir to combine.

5. Cover pot with lid and cook on high pressure for 35 minutes.

6. When finished, allow to release pressure naturally then open the lid.

7. Stir well and serve.

Nutrition: Calories 276; Fat 4.8 g; Carbohydrates 44.2 g; Sugar 2.3 g; Protein 16.6 g; Cholesterol 0 mg

Kale Cauliflower Soup

Preparation Time: 10 minutes

Cooking Time: 25 minutes

Servings: 4

Ingredients:

- 2 cups baby kale
- ½ cup unsweetened coconut milk
- 4 cups of water
- 1 large cauliflower head, chopped
- 3 garlic cloves, peeled
- 2 carrots, peeled and chopped
- 2 onion, chopped
- 3 tbsp. olive oil
- Pepper
- Salt

Directions:

1. Add oil into the instant pot and set the pot on sauté mode.

2. Add carrot, garlic, and onion to the pot and sauté for 5-7 minutes.

3. Add water and cauliflower and stir well.

4. Cover pot with lid and cook on high pressure for 20 minutes.

5. When finished, release pressure using the quick release **Directions:** than open the lid.

6. Add kale and coconut milk and stir well.

7. Blend the soup utilizing a submersion blender until smooth.

8. Season with pepper and salt.

Nutrition: Calories 261; Fat 18.1 g; Carbohydrates 23.9 g; Sugar 9.9 g; Protein 6.6 g; Cholesterol 0 mg

Healthy Broccoli Asparagus Soup

Preparation Time: 10 minutes

Cooking Time: 20 minutes

Servings: 6

Ingredients:

- 2 cups broccoli florets, chopped
- 15 asparagus spear, ends trimmed and chopped
- 1 tsp. dried oregano
- 1 tbsp. fresh thyme leaves
- ½ cup unsweetened almond milk
- 3 ½ cups filtered alkaline water
- 2 cups cauliflower florets, chopped
- 2 tsp. garlic, chopped
- 1 cup onion, chopped
- 2 tbsp. olive oil

- Pepper
- Salt

Directions:

1. Add oil in the instant pot and set the pot on sauté mode.

2. Add onion to the olive oil and sauté until onion is softened.

3. Add garlic and sauté for 30 seconds.

4. Add all vegetables and water and stir well.

5. Cover pot with lid and cook on manual mode for 3 minutes.

6. When finished, allow to release pressure naturally then open the lid.

7. Blend the soup utilizing a submersion blender until smooth.

8. Stir in almond milk, herbs, pepper, and salt.

9. Serve and enjoy.

Nutrition: Calories 85; Fat 5.2 g; Carbohydrates 8.8 g; Sugar 3.3 g; Protein 3.3 g; Cholesterol 0 mg

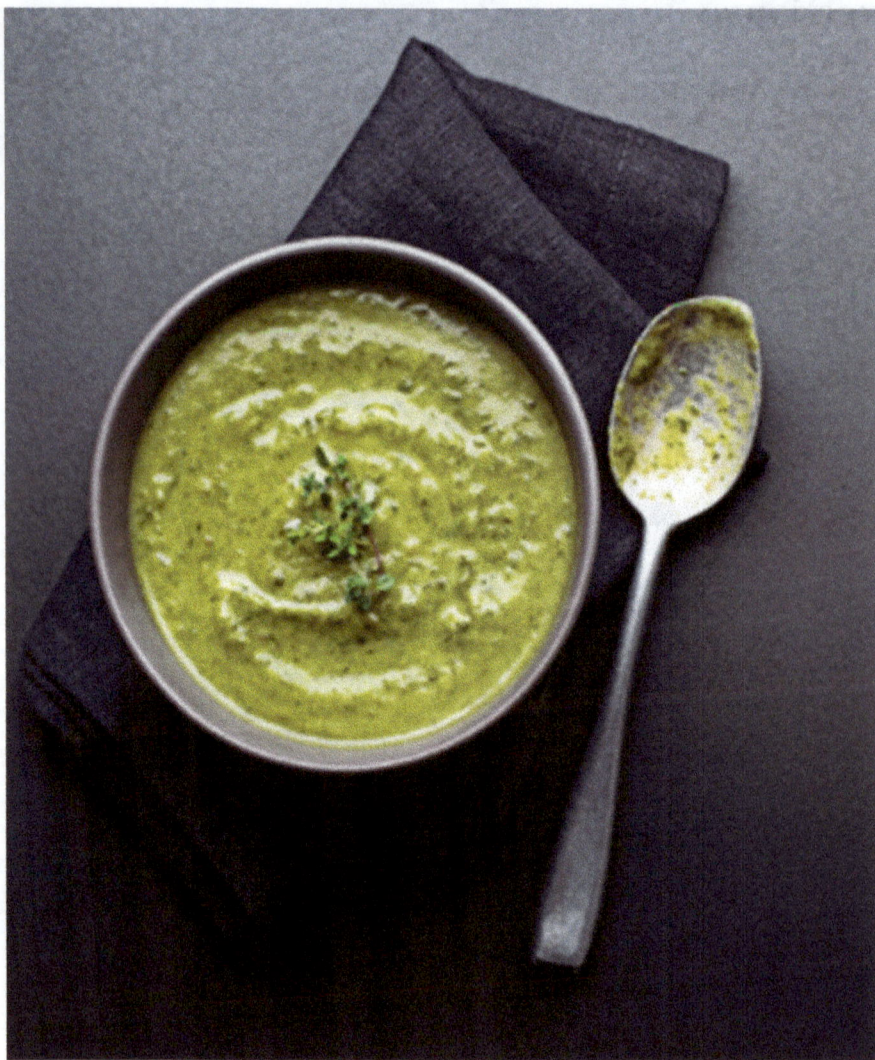

Creamy Asparagus Soup

Preparation Time: 10 minutes

Cooking Time: 30 minutes

Servings: 6

Ingredients:

- 2 lbs. fresh asparagus cut off woody stems

- ¼ tsp. lime zest

- 2 tbsp. lime juice

- 14 oz. coconut milk

- 1 tsp. dried thyme

- ½ tsp. oregano

- ½ tsp. sage

- 1 ½ cups filtered alkaline water

- 1 cauliflower head, cut into florets

- 1 tbsp. garlic, minced

- 1 leek, sliced

- 3 tbsp. coconut oil

- Pinch of Himalayan salt

Directions:

- Preheat the oven to 400 F/ 200 C.

- Line baking tray with parchment paper and set aside.

- Arrange asparagus spears on a baking tray. Drizzle with 2 tablespoons of coconut oil and sprinkle with salt, thyme, oregano, and sage.

- Bake in preheated oven for 20-25 minutes.

- Add remaining oil in the instant pot and set the pot on sauté mode.

- Put some garlic and leek to the pot and sauté for 2-3 minutes.

- Add cauliflower florets and water in the pot and stir well.

- Cover pot with lid and select steam mode and set timer for 4 minutes.

- When finished, release pressure using the quick release **Directions** .

- Add roasted asparagus, lime zest, lime juice, and coconut milk and stir well.

- Blend the soup utilizing a submersion blender until smooth.

- Serve and enjoy.

Nutrition: Calories 265; Fat 22.9 g; Carbohydrates 14.7 g; Sugar 6.7 g; Protein 6.1 g; Cholesterol 0 mg

Quick Broccoli Soup

Preparation Time: 5 minutes

Cooking Time: 10 minutes

Servings: 6

Ingredients:

- 1 lb. broccoli, chopped
- 6 cups filtered alkaline water
- 1 onion, diced
- 2 tbsp. olive oil
- Pepper
- Salt

Directions:

1. Add oil into the instant pot and set the pot on sauté mode.

2. Add onion in olive oil and sauté until softened.

3. Add broccoli and water and stir well.

4. Cover pot with top and cook on manual high pressure for 3 minutes.

5. When finished, release pressure using the quick release **Directions:** than open the lid.

6. Blend the soup utilizing a submersion blender until smooth.

7. Season soup with pepper and salt.

8. Serve and enjoy.

Nutrition: Calories 73; Fat 4.9 g; Carbohydrates 6.7 g; Protein 2.3 g; Sugar 2.1 g; Cholesterol 0 mg

Green Lentil Soup

Preparation Time: 10 minutes

Cooking Time: 30 minutes

Servings: 4

Ingredients:

- 1 ½ cups green lentils, rinsed
- 4 cups baby spinach
- 4 cups filtered alkaline water
- 1 tsp. Italian seasoning
- 2 tsp. fresh thyme
- 14 oz. tomatoes, diced
- 3 garlic cloves, minced
- 2 celery stalks, chopped
- 1 carrot, chopped
- 1 onion, chopped
- Pepper

- Sea salt

Directions:

1. Add all **Ingredients** except spinach into the direct pot and mix fine.

2. Cover pot with top and cook on manual high pressure for 18 minutes.

3. When finished, release pressure using the quick release **Directions:** than open the lid.

4. Add spinach and stir well.

5. Serve and enjoy.

__Nutrition:__ Calories 306; Fat 1.5 g; Carbohydrates 53.7 g; Sugar 6.4 g; Protein 21 g; Cholesterol 1 mg

Squash Soup

Preparation Time: 10 minutes

Cooking Time: 40 minutes

Servings: 4

Ingredients:

- 3 lbs. butternut squash, peeled and cubed
- 1 tbsp. curry powder
- 1/2 cup unsweetened coconut milk
- 3 cups filtered alkaline water
- 2 garlic cloves, minced
- 1 large onion, minced
- 1 tsp. olive oil

Directions:

1. Add olive oil in the instant pot and set the pot on sauté mode.

2. Add onion and cook until tender, about 8 minutes.

3. Add curry powder and garlic and sauté for a minute.

4. Add butternut squash, water, and salt and stir well.

5. Cover pot with lid and cook on soup mode for 30 minutes.

6. When finished, allow to release pressure naturally for 10 minutes then release using quick release **Directions:** than open the lid.

7. Blend the soup utilizing a submersion blender until smooth.

8. Add coconut milk and stir well.

9. Serve warm and enjoy.

Nutrition: Calories 254; Fat 8.9 g; Carbohydrates 46.4 g; Sugar 10.1 g; Protein 4.8 g; Cholesterol 0 mg

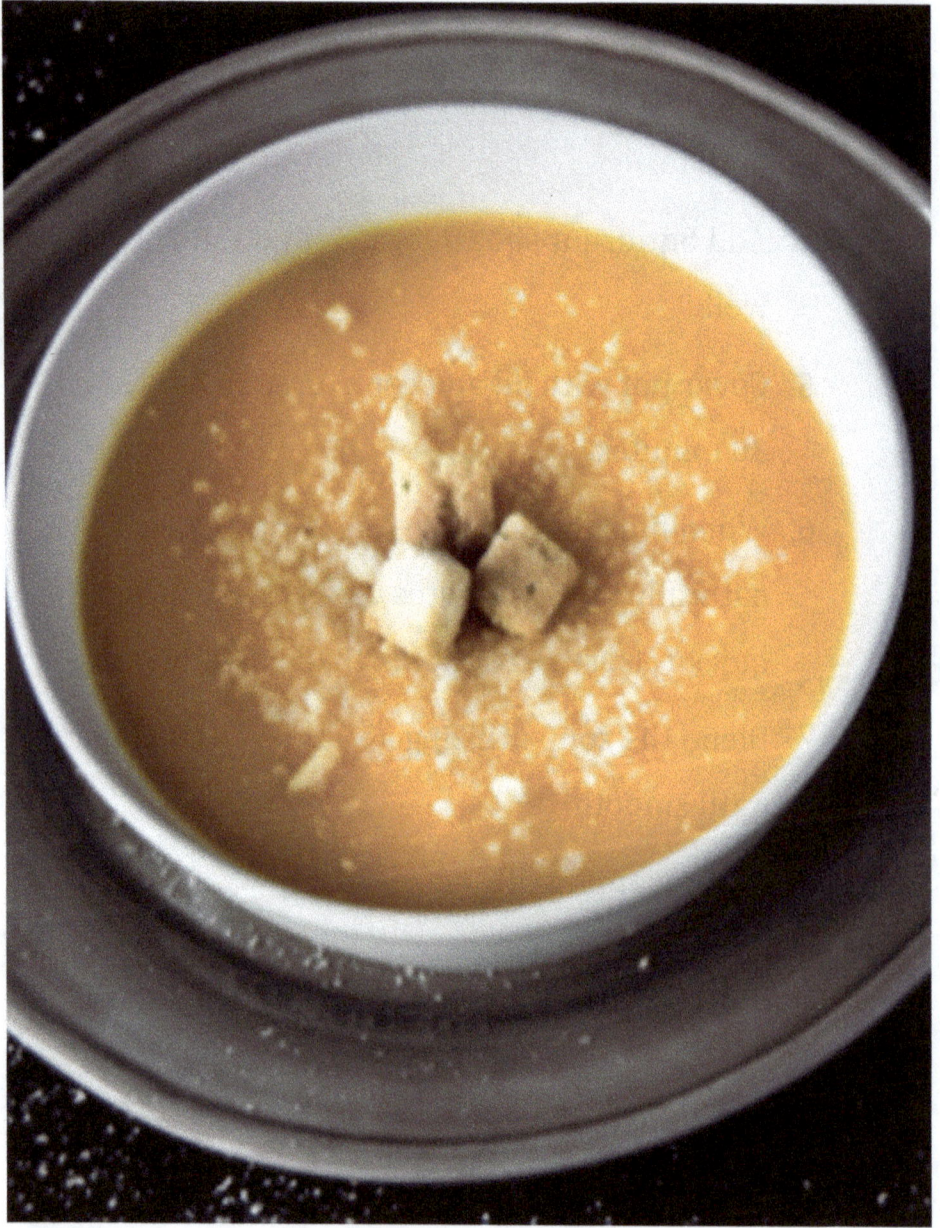

Tomato Soup

Preparation Time: 5 minutes

Cooking Time: 20 minutes

Servings: 4

Ingredients:

- 6 tomatoes, chopped

- 1 onion, diced

- 14 oz. coconut milk

- 1 tsp. turmeric

- 1 tsp. garlic, minced

- 1/4 cup cilantro, chopped

- 1/2 tsp. cayenne pepper

- 1 tsp. ginger, minced

- 1/2 tsp. sea salt

Directions:

1. Add all Ingredients to the direct pot and mix fine.

2. Cover instant pot with lid and cook on manual high pressure for 5 minutes.

3. When finished, allow to release pressure naturally for 10 minutes then release using the quick release Directions

4. Blend the soup utilizing a submersion blender until smooth.

5. Stir well and serve.

__Nutrition:__ Calories 81; Fat 3.5 g; Carbohydrates 11.6 g; Sugar 6.1 g; Protein 2.5 g; Cholesterol 0 mg

Basil Zucchini Soup

Preparation Time: 10 minutes

Cooking Time: 20 minutes

Servings: 4

Ingredients:

- 3 medium zucchinis, peeled and chopped
- 1/4 cup basil, chopped
- 1 large leek, chopped
- 3 cups filtered alkaline water
- 1 tbsp. lemon juice
- 3 tbsp. olive oil
- 2 tsp. sea salt

Directions:

1. Add 2 tbsp. oil into the pot and set the pot on sauté mode.

2. Add zucchini and sauté for 5 minutes.

3. Add basil and leeks and sauté for 2-3 minutes.

4. Add lemon juice, water, and salt. Stir well.

5. Cover pot with lid and cook on high pressure for 8 minutes.

6. When finished, allow to release pressure naturally then open the lid.

7. Blend the soup utilizing a submersion blender until smooth.

8. Top with remaining olive oil and serve.

Nutrition: Calories 157; Fat 11.9 g; Carbohydrates 8.9 g; Protein 5.8 g; Sugar 4 g; Cholesterol 0 mg

Summer Vegetable Soup

Preparation Time: 5 minutes

Cooking Time: 20 minutes

Servings: 10

Ingredients:

- 1/2 cup basil, chopped
- 2 bell peppers, seeded and sliced
- 1/ cup green beans, trimmed and cut into pieces
- 8 cups filtered alkaline water
- 1 medium summer squash, sliced
- 1 medium zucchini, sliced
- 2 large tomatoes, sliced
- 1 small eggplant, sliced
- 6 garlic cloves, smashed
- 1 medium onion, diced

- Pepper
- Salt

Directions:

1. Combine all elements into the direct pot and mix fine.

2. Cover pot with lid and cook on soup mode for 10 minutes.

3. Release pressure using quick release **Directions:** than open the lid.

4. Blend the soup utilizing a submersion blender until smooth.

5. Serve and enjoy.

__Nutrition:__ Calories 84; Fat 1.6 g; Carbohydrates 12.8 g; Protein 6.1 g; Sugar 6.1 g; Cholesterol 0 mg

Almond-Red Bell Pepper Dip

Preparation Time: 14 minutes

Cooking Time: 16 minutes

Servings: *3*

Ingredients:

- Garlic, 2-3 cloves

- Sea salt, one (1) pinch

- Cayenne pepper, one (1) pinch

- Extra virgin olive oil (cold pressed), one (1) tablespoon

- Almonds, 60g

- Red bell pepper, 280g

Directions:

1. First of all, cook garlic and pepper until they are soft.

2. Add all **Ingredients** in a mixer and blend until the mix becomes smooth and creamy.

3. Finally, add pepper and salt to taste.

4. Serve.

Nutrition: Calories: 51; Carbohydrates: 10g; Fat: 1g; Protein: 2g

Spicy Carrot Soup

Preparation Time: 10 minutes

Cooking Time: 20 minutes

Servings: 6

Ingredients:

- 8 large carrots, peeled and chopped
- 1 1/2 cups filtered alkaline water
- 14 oz. coconut milk
- 3 garlic cloves, peeled
- 1 tbsp. red curry paste
- 1/4 cup olive oil
- 1 onion, chopped
- Salt

Directions:

1. Combine all elements into the direct pot and mix fine.

2. Cover pot with lid and select manual and set timer for 15 minutes.

3. Allow to release pressure naturally then open the lid.

4. Blend the soup utilizing a submersion blender until smooth.

5. Serve and enjoy.

Nutrition: Calories 267; Fat 22 g; Carbohydrates 13 g; Protein 4 g; Sugar 5 g; Cholesterol 20 mg

Zucchini Soup

Preparation Time: 10 minutes

Cooking Time: 30 minutes

Servings: *10*

Ingredients:

- 10 cups zucchini, chopped
- 32 oz. filtered alkaline water
- 13.5 oz. coconut milk
- 1 tbsp. Thai curry paste

Directions:

1. Combine all elements into the direct pot and mix fine.
2. Cover pot with lid and cook on manual high pressure for 10 minutes.
3. Release pressure using quick release Directions then open the lid.
4. Using blender Blend the soup until smooth.

5. Serve and enjoy.

Nutrition: Calories 122; Fat 9.8 g; Carbohydrates 6.6 g; Protein 4.1 g; Sugar 3.6 g; Cholesterol 0 mg

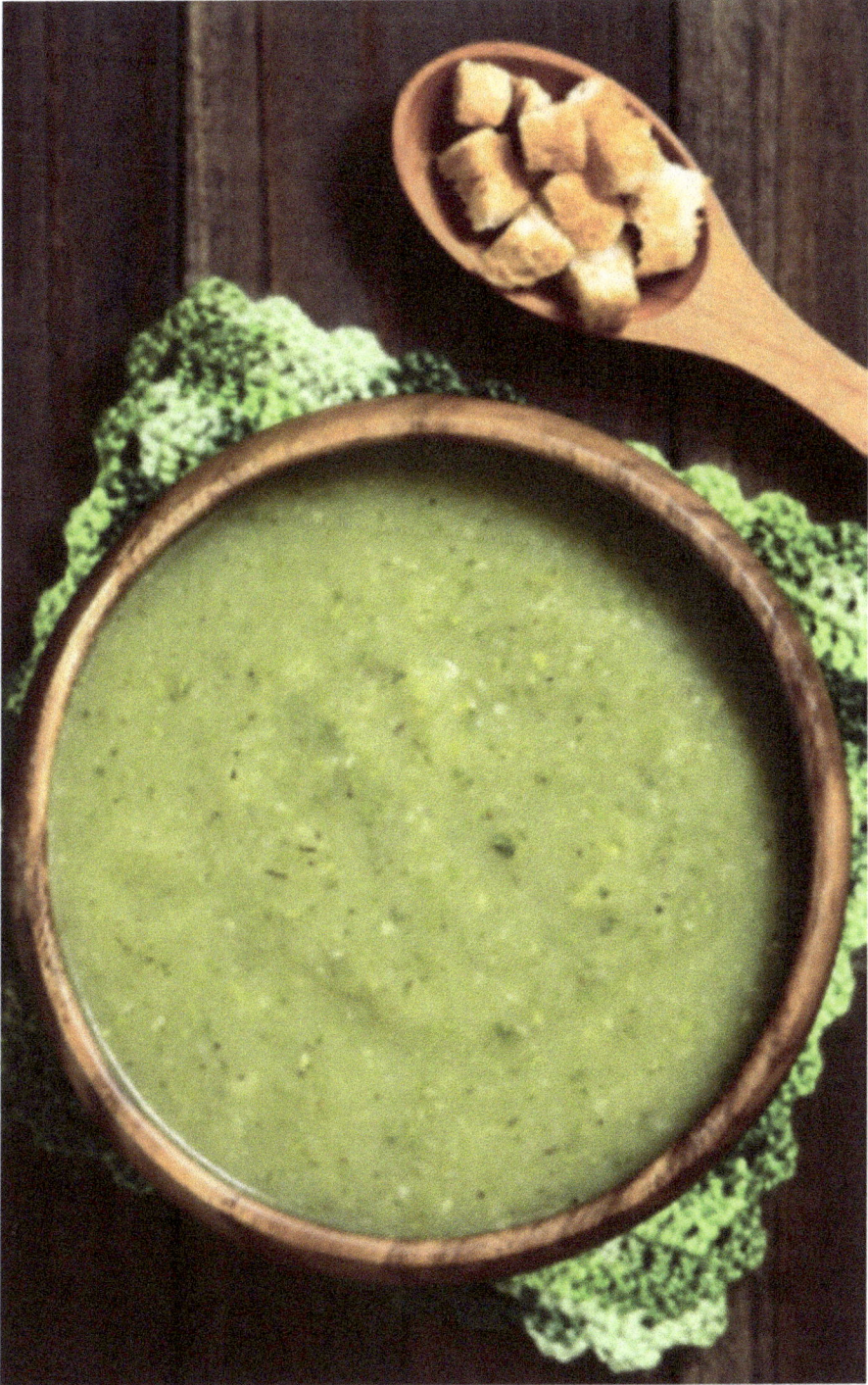

Kidney Bean Stew

Preparation Time: 15 minutes

Cooking Time: 15 minutes

Servings: *2*

Ingredients:

- 1lb cooked kidney beans

- 1 cup tomato passata

- 1 cup low sodium beef broth

- 3tbsp Italian herbs

Directions:

1. Mix all the **Ingredients** in your Instant Pot.

2. Cook on Stew for 15 minutes.

3. Release the pressure naturally.

Nutrition: Calories: 270; Carbs: 16; Sugar: 3; Fat: 10; Protein: 23; GL: 8

Cabbage Soup

Preparation Time: 15 minutes

Cooking Time: 35 minutes

Servings: *2*

Ingredients:

- 1lb shredded cabbage

- 1 cup low sodium vegetable broth

- 1 shredded onion

- 2tbsp mixed herbs

- 1tbsp black pepper

Recipe*:*

1. Mix all the **Ingredients** in your Instant Pot.

2. Cook on Stew for 35 minutes.

3. Release the pressure naturally.

Nutrition: Calories: 60; Carbs: 2; Sugar: 0; Fat: 2; Protein: 4; GL: 1

Pumpkin Spice Soup

Preparation Time: 10 minutes

Cooking Time: 35 minutes

Servings: *2*

Ingredients:

- 1lb cubed pumpkin
- 1 cup low sodium vegetable broth
- 2tbsp mixed spice

Recipe:

1. Mix all the **Ingredients** in your Instant Pot.
2. Cook on Stew for 35 minutes.
3. Release the pressure naturally.
4. Blend the soup.

Nutrition: Calories: 100; Carbs: 7; Sugar: 1; Fat: 2; Protein: 3; GL: 1

Cream of Tomato Soup

Preparation Time: 15 minutes

Cooking Time: 15 minutes

Servings: *2*

Ingredients:

- 1lb fresh tomatoes, chopped

- 1.5 cups low sodium tomato puree

- 1tbsp black pepper

Directions:

1. Mix all the **Ingredients** in your Instant Pot.

2. Cook on Stew for 15 minutes.

3. Release the pressure naturally.

4. Blend.

Nutrition: Calories: 20; Carbs: 2; Sugar: 1; Fat: 0; Protein: 3; GL: 1

Shiitake Soup

Preparation Time: 15 minutes

Cooking Time: 35 minutes

Servings: *2*

Ingredients:

- 1 cup shiitake mushrooms
- 1 cup diced vegetables
- 1 cup low sodium vegetable broth
- 2tbsp 5 spice seasoning

Directions:

1. Mix all the **Ingredients** in your Instant Pot.
2. Cook on Stew for 35 minutes.
3. Release the pressure naturally.

Nutrition: Calories: 70; Carbs: 5; Sugar: 1; Fat: 2; Protein: 2; GL: 1

Spicy Pepper Soup

Preparation Time: 15 minutes

Cooking Time: 15 minutes

Servings: *2*

Ingredients:

- 1lb chopped mixed sweet peppers
- 1 cup low sodium vegetable broth
- 3tbsp chopped chili peppers
- 1tbsp black pepper

Directions:

1. Mix all the **Ingredients** in your Instant Pot.
2. Cook on Stew for 15 minutes.
3. Release the pressure naturally. Blend.

Nutrition: Calories: 100; Carbs: 11; Sugar: 4; Fat: 2; Protein: 3; GL: 6

Zoodle Won-Ton Soup

Preparation Time: 15 minutes

Cooking Time: 5 minutes

Servings: *2*

Ingredients:

- 1lb spiralized zucchini

- 1 pack unfried won-tons

- 1 cup low sodium beef broth

- 2tbsp soy sauce

Directions:

1. Mix all the **Ingredients** in your Instant Pot.

2. Cook on Stew for 5 minutes.

3. Release the pressure naturally.

Nutrition: Calories: 300; Carbs: 6; Sugar: 1; Fat: 9; Protein: 43; GL: 2

Broccoli Stilton Soup

Preparation Time: 15 minutes

Cooking Time: 35 minutes

Servings: *2*

Ingredients:

- 1lb chopped broccoli
- 0.5lb chopped vegetables
- 1 cup low sodium vegetable broth
- 1 cup Stilton

Directions:

1. Mix all the **Ingredients** in your Instant Pot.
2. Cook on Stew for 35 minutes.
3. Release the pressure naturally.
4. Blend the soup.

Nutrition: Calories: 280; Carbs: 9; Sugar: 2; Fat: 22;

Protein: 13; GL: 4

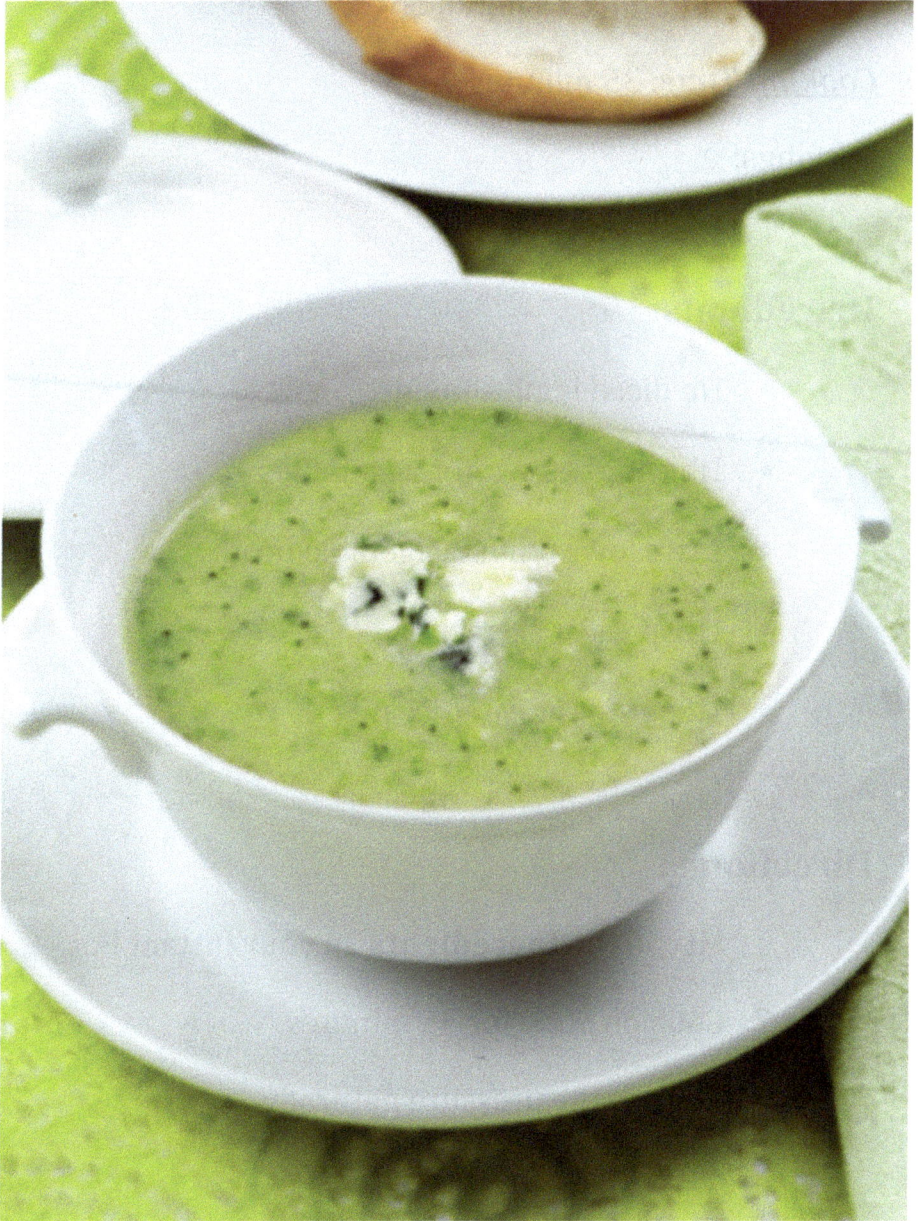

Lamb Stew

__Preparation Time:__ 15 minutes

__Cooking Time__: 35 minutes

Servings: *2*

Ingredients:

- 1lb diced lamb shoulder
- 1lb chopped winter vegetables
- 1 cup low sodium vegetable broth
- 1tbsp yeast extract
- 1tbsp star anise spice mix

Directions:

1. Mix all the **Ingredients** in your Instant Pot.
2. Cook on Stew for 35 minutes.
3. Release the pressure naturally.

Nutrition: Calories: 320; Carbs: 10; Sugar: 2; Fat: 8; Protein: 42; GL: 3

Irish Stew

Preparation Time: 15 minutes

Cooking Time: 35 minutes

Servings: *2*

Ingredients:

- 1.5lb diced lamb shoulder
- 1lb chopped vegetables
- 1 cup low sodium beef broth
- 3 minced onions
- 1tbsp ghee

Directions:

1. Mix all the **Ingredients** in your Instant Pot.
2. Cook on Stew for 35 minutes.
3. Release the pressure naturally.

Nutrition: Calories: 330; Carbs: 9; Sugar: 2; Fat: 12; Protein: 49; GL: 3

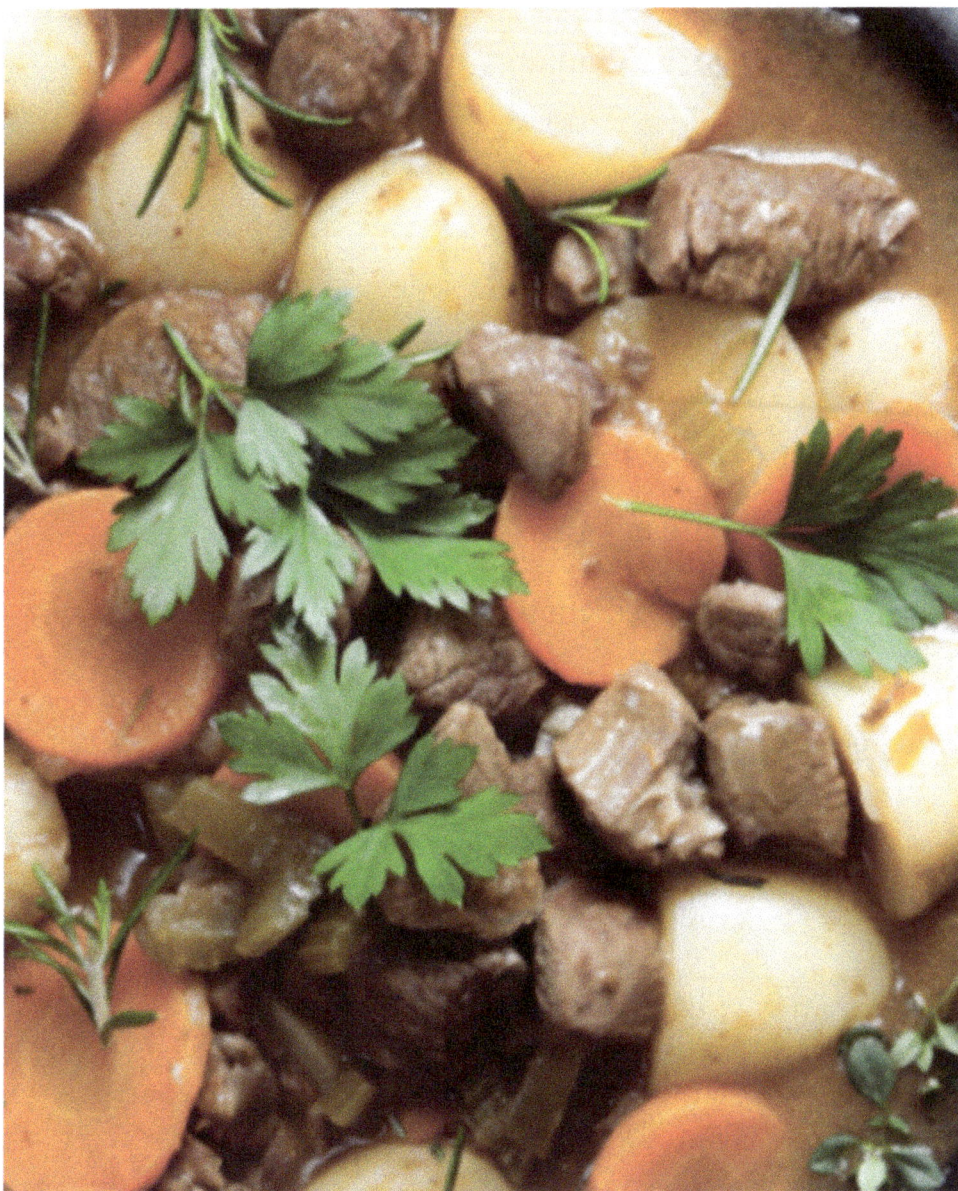

Sweet and Sour Soup

Preparation Time: 15 minutes

Cooking Time: 35 minutes

Servings: *2*

Ingredients:

- 1lb cubed chicken breast
- 1lb chopped vegetables
- 1 cup low carb sweet and sour sauce
- 0.5 cup diabetic marmalade

Directions:

1. Mix all the Ingredients in your Instant Pot.
2. Cook on Stew for 35 minutes.
3. Release the pressure naturally.

Meatball Stew

Preparation Time: 15 minutes

Cooking Time: 25 minutes

Servings: *2*

Ingredients:

- 1lb sausage meat
- 2 cups chopped tomato
- 1 cup chopped vegetables
- 2tbsp Italian seasonings
- 1tbsp vegetable oil

Directions:

1. Roll the sausage into meatballs.
2. Put the Instant Pot on Sauté and fry the meatballs in the oil until brown.
3. Mix all the Ingredients in your Instant Pot.
4. Cook on Stew for 25 minutes.

5. Release the pressure naturally.

Nutrition: Calories: 300; Carbs: 4; Sugar: 1; Fat: 12; Protein: 40; GL: 2

Kebab Stew

__Preparation Time:__ 15 minutes

__Cooking Time__: 35 minutes

Servings: *2*

Ingredients:

- 1lb cubed, seasoned kebab meat

- 1lb cooked chickpeas

- 1 cup low sodium vegetable broth

- 1tbsp black pepper

Directions:

1. Mix all the **Ingredients** in your Instant Pot.

2. Cook on Stew for 35 minutes.

3. Release the pressure naturally.

__Nutrition:__ Calories: 290; Carbs: 22; Sugar: 4; Fat: 10; Protein: 34; GL: 6

French Onion Soup

Preparation Time: 35 minutes

Cooking Time: 35 minutes

Servings: *2*

Ingredients:

- 6 onions, chopped finely
- 2 cups vegetable broth
- 2tbsp oil
- 2tbsp Gruyere

Directions:

1. Place the oil in your Instant Pot and cook the onions on Sauté until soft and brown.
2. Mix all the Ingredients in your Instant Pot.
3. Cook on Stew for 35 minutes.
4. Release the pressure naturally.

Nutrition: Calories: 110; Carbs: 8; Sugar: 3; Fat: 10;

Protein: 3; GL: 4

Meatless Ball Soup

Preparation Time: 15 minutes

Cooking Time: 15 minutes

Servings: *2*

Ingredients:

- 1lb minced tofu
- 0.5lb chopped vegetables
- 2 cups low sodium vegetable broth
- 1tbsp almond flour
- salt and pepper

Directions:

1. Mix the tofu, flour, salt and pepper.
2. Form the meatballs.
3. Place all the Ingredients in your Instant Pot.
4. Cook on Stew for 15 minutes.
5. Release the pressure naturally.

__Nutrition:__ Calories: 240; Carbs: 9; Sugar: 3; Fat: 10; Protein: 35; GL: 5

Fake-On Stew

Preparation Time: 15 minutes

Cooking Time: 25 minutes

Servings: *2*

Ingredients:

- 0.5lb soy bacon
- 1lb chopped vegetables
- 1 cup low sodium vegetable broth
- 1tbsp Nutritional yeast
-

Directions:

1. Mix all the **Ingredients** in your Instant Pot.
2. Cook on Stew for 25 minutes.
3. Release the pressure naturally.

Nutrition: Calories: 200; Carbs: 12; Sugar: 3; Fat: 7; Protein: 41; GL: 5

Chickpea Soup

Preparation Time: 15 minutes

Cooking Time: 35 minutes

Servings: *2*

Ingredients:

- 1lb cooked chickpeas
- 1lb chopped vegetables
- 1 cup low sodium vegetable broth
- 2tbsp mixed herbs

Directions:

1. Mix all the **Ingredients** in your Instant Pot.
2. Cook on Stew for 35 minutes.
3. Release the pressure naturally.

Nutrition: Calories: 310; Carbs: 20; Sugar: 3; Fat: 5; Protein: 27; GL: 5

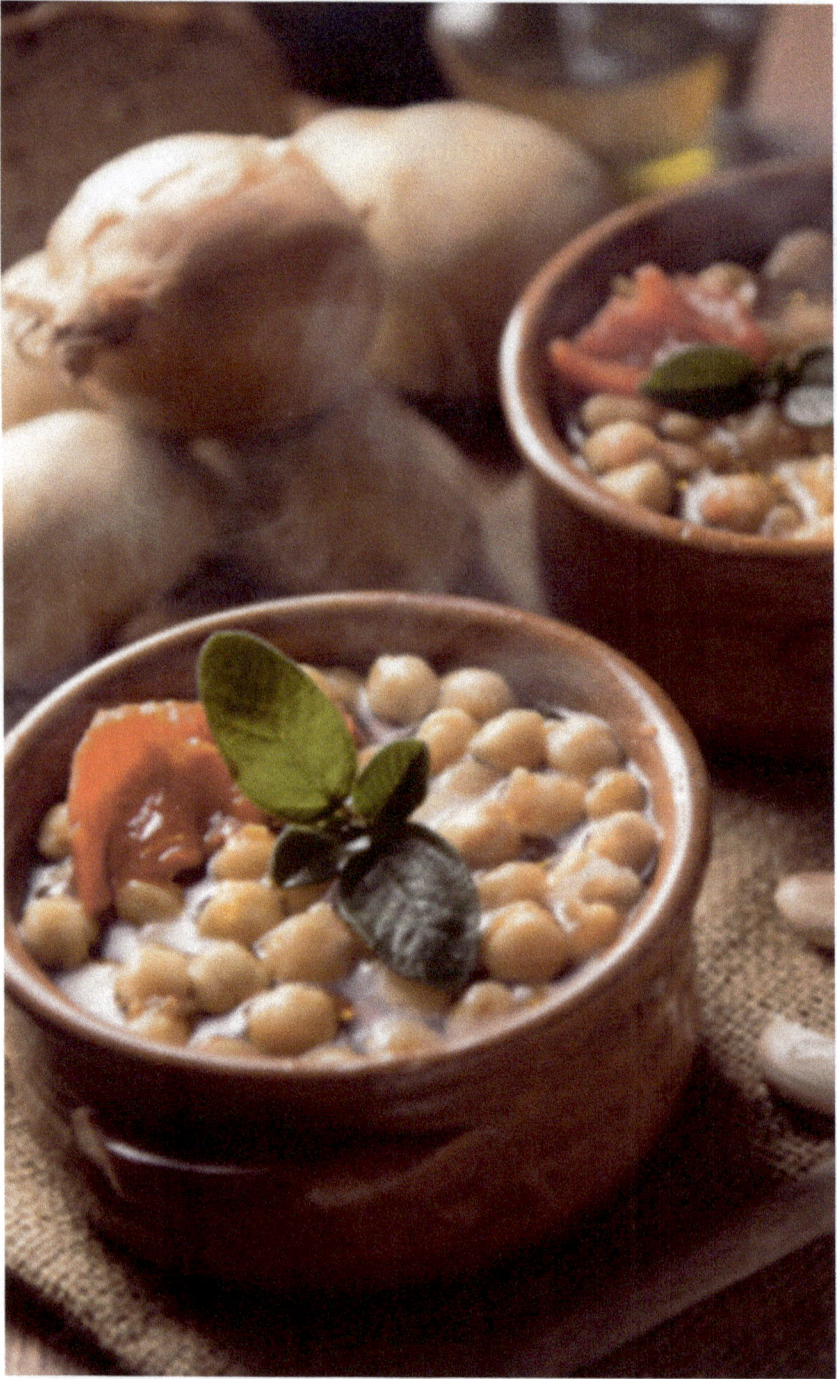

Chicken Zoodle Soup

Preparation Time: 15 minutes

Cooking Time: 35 minutes

Servings: *2*

Ingredients:

- 1lb chopped cooked chicken
- 1lb spiralized zucchini
- 1 cup low sodium chicken soup
- 1 cup diced vegetables

Directions:

1. Mix all the ingredients except the zucchini in your Instant Pot.
2. Cook on Stew for 35 minutes.
3. Release the pressure naturally.
4. Stir in the zucchini and allow to heat thoroughly.

Nutrition: Calories: 250; Carbs: 5; Sugar: 0; Fat: 10;

Protein: 40; GL: 1

Lemon-Tarragon Soup

Preparation Time: 10 minutes

Cooking Time: 10 minutes

Servings: 1-2

Cashews and coconut milk replace heavy cream in this healthy version of lemon-tarragon soup, balanced by tart freshly squeezed lemon juice and fragrant tarragon. It's a light, airy soup that you won't want to miss.

Ingredients:

- 1 tablespoon avocado oil
- ½ cup diced onion
- 3 garlic cloves, crushed
- ¼ plus 1/8 teaspoon sea salt
- ¼ plus 1/8 teaspoon freshly ground black pepper
- 1 (13.5-ounce) can full-fat coconut milk
- 1 tablespoon freshly squeezed lemon juice

- ½ cup raw cashews

- 1 celery stalk

- 2 tablespoons chopped fresh tarragon

Directions:

1. In a medium skillet over medium-high warmth, heat the avocado oil. Add the onion, garlic, salt, and pepper, and sauté for 3 to 5 minutes or until the onion is soft.

2. In a high-speed blender, blend together the coconut milk, lemon juice, cashews, celery, and tarragon with the onion mixture until smooth. Adjust seasonings, if necessary.

3. Fill 1 huge or 2 little dishes and enjoy immediately, or transfer to a medium saucepan and warm on low heat for 3 to 5 minutes before serving.

Nutrition: Calories: 60; Carbohydrates: 13 g;Protein: 0.8 g

Chilled Cucumber and Lime Soup

Preparation Time: 5 minutes

Cooking Time: 20 minutes

Servings: 1-2

Ingredients:

- 1 cucumber, peeled

- ½ zucchini, peeled

- 1 tablespoon freshly squeezed lime juice

- 1 tablespoon fresh cilantro leaves

- 1 garlic clove, crushed

- ¼ teaspoon sea salt

Directions:

1. In a blender, blend together the cucumber, zucchini, lime juice, cilantro, garlic, and salt until well combined. Add more salt, if necessary.

2. Fill 1 huge or 2 little dishes and enjoy immediately, or refrigerate for 15 to 20 minutes to chill before serving.

Nutrition: Calories: 48; Carbohydrates: 8 g; Fat: 1g; Protein: 5g

Coconut, Cilantro, And Jalapeño Soup

Preparation Time: 5 minutes

Cooking Time: 5 minutes

Servings: 1-2

This soup is a nutrient dream. Cilantro is a natural anti-inflammatory and is also excellent for detoxification. And one single jalapeño has an entire day's worth of vitamin C!

Ingredients:

- 2 tablespoons avocado oil

- ½ cup diced onions

- 3 garlic cloves, crushed

- ¼ teaspoon sea salt

- 1 (13.5-ounce) can full-fat coconut milk

- 1 tablespoon freshly squeezed lime juice

- ½ to 1 jalapeño

- 2 tablespoons fresh cilantro leaves

Directions:

1. In a medium skillet over medium-high warmth, heat the avocado oil. Include the garlic, onion salt, and pepper, and sauté for 3 to 5 minutes, or until the onions are soft.

2. In a blender, blend together the coconut milk, lime juice, jalapeño, and cilantro with the onion mixture until creamy.

3. Fill 1 huge or 2 little dishes and enjoy.

Nutrition: Calories: 75; Carbohydrates: 13 g; Fat: 2 g; Protein: 4 g

Spicy Watermelon Gazpacho

__Preparation Time:__ 5 minutes

__Cooking Time__: 5 minutes

__Servings:__ 1-2

At first taste, this soup may have you wondering if you're lunching on a hot and spicy salsa. It has the heat and seasonings of a traditional tomato-based salsa, but it also has a faint sweetness from the cool watermelon. The soup is really hot with a whole jalapeño, so if you don't like food too hot, just use half a jalapeño.

__Ingredients:__

- 2 cups cubed watermelon
- ¼ cup diced onion
- ¼ cup packed cilantro leaves
- ½ to 1 jalapeño
- 2 tablespoons freshly squeezed lime juice

Directions:

1. In a blender or food processor, pulse to combine the watermelon, onion, cilantro, jalapeño, and lime juice only long enough to break down the **Ingredients** , leaving them very finely diced and taking care to not over process.

2. Pour into 1 large or 2 small bowls and enjoy.

Nutrition: Calories: 35; Carbohydrates: 12; Fat: 4 g

Roasted Carrot and Leek Soup

Preparation Time: 4 minutes

Cooking Time: 30 minutes

Servings: 3-4

The carrot, a root vegetable, is an excellent source of antioxidants (1 cup has 113 percent of your daily value of vitamin A) and fiber (1 cup has 14 percent of your daily value). This bright and colorful soup freezes well to enjoy later when you're short on time.

Ingredients:

- 6 carrots
- 1 cup chopped onion
- 1 fennel bulb, cubed
- 2 garlic cloves, crushed
- 2 tablespoons avocado oil
- 1 teaspoon sea salt
- 1 teaspoon freshly ground black pepper

- 2 cups almond milk, plus more if desired

Directions:

1. Preheat the oven to 400°F. Line a baking sheet with parchment paper.

2. Cut the carrots into thirds, and then cut each third in half. Transfer to a medium bowl.

3. Add the onion, fennel, garlic, and avocado oil, and toss to coat. Season with the salt and pepper, and toss again.

4. Transfer the vegetables to the prepared baking sheet, and roast for 30 minutes.

5. Remove from the oven and allow the vegetables to cool.

6. In a high-speed blender, blend together the almond milk and roasted vegetables until creamy and smooth. Adjust the seasonings, if necessary, and add additional milk if you prefer a thinner consistency.

7. Pour into 2 large or 4 small bowls and enjoy.

Nutrition: Calories: 55; Carbohydrates: 12g; Fat: 1.5 g; Protein: 1.8 g

Creamy Lentil and Potato Stew

Preparation Time: 10 minutes

Cooking Time: 30 minutes

Servings: 4

This is a hearty stew that is sure to be a favorite. It's a one-pot meal that is the perfect comfort food. With fresh vegetables and herbs along with protein-rich lentils, it's both healthy and filling. Any lentil variety would work, even a mixed, sprouted lentil blend. Another bonus of this recipe: It's freezer-friendly.

Ingredients:

- 2 tablespoons avocado oil
- ½ cup diced onion
- 2 garlic cloves, crushed
- 1 to 1½ teaspoons sea salt
- 1 teaspoon freshly ground black pepper
- 1 cup dry lentils

- 2 carrots, sliced

- 1 cup peeled and cubed potato

- 1 celery stalk, diced

- 2 fresh oregano sprigs, chopped

- 2 fresh tarragon sprigs, chopped

- 5 cups vegetable broth, divided

- 1 (13.5-ounce) can full-fat coconut milk

Directions:

1. In a great soup pot over average-high hotness, heat the avocado oil. Include the garlic, onion, salt, and pepper, and sauté for 3 to 5 minutes, or until the onion is soft.

2. Add the lentils, carrots, potato, celery, oregano, tarragon, and 2½ cups of vegetable broth, and stir.

3. Get to a boil, decrease the heat to medium-low, and cook, stirring frequently and adding additional vegetable broth a half cup at a time

to make sure there is enough liquid for the lentils and potatoes to cook, for 20 to 25 minutes, or until the potatoes and lentils are soft.

4. Take away from the heat, and stirring in the coconut milk. Pour into 4 soup bowls and enjoy.

Nutrition: Calories: 85; Carbohydrates: 20g; Fat: 3g; Protein: 3g

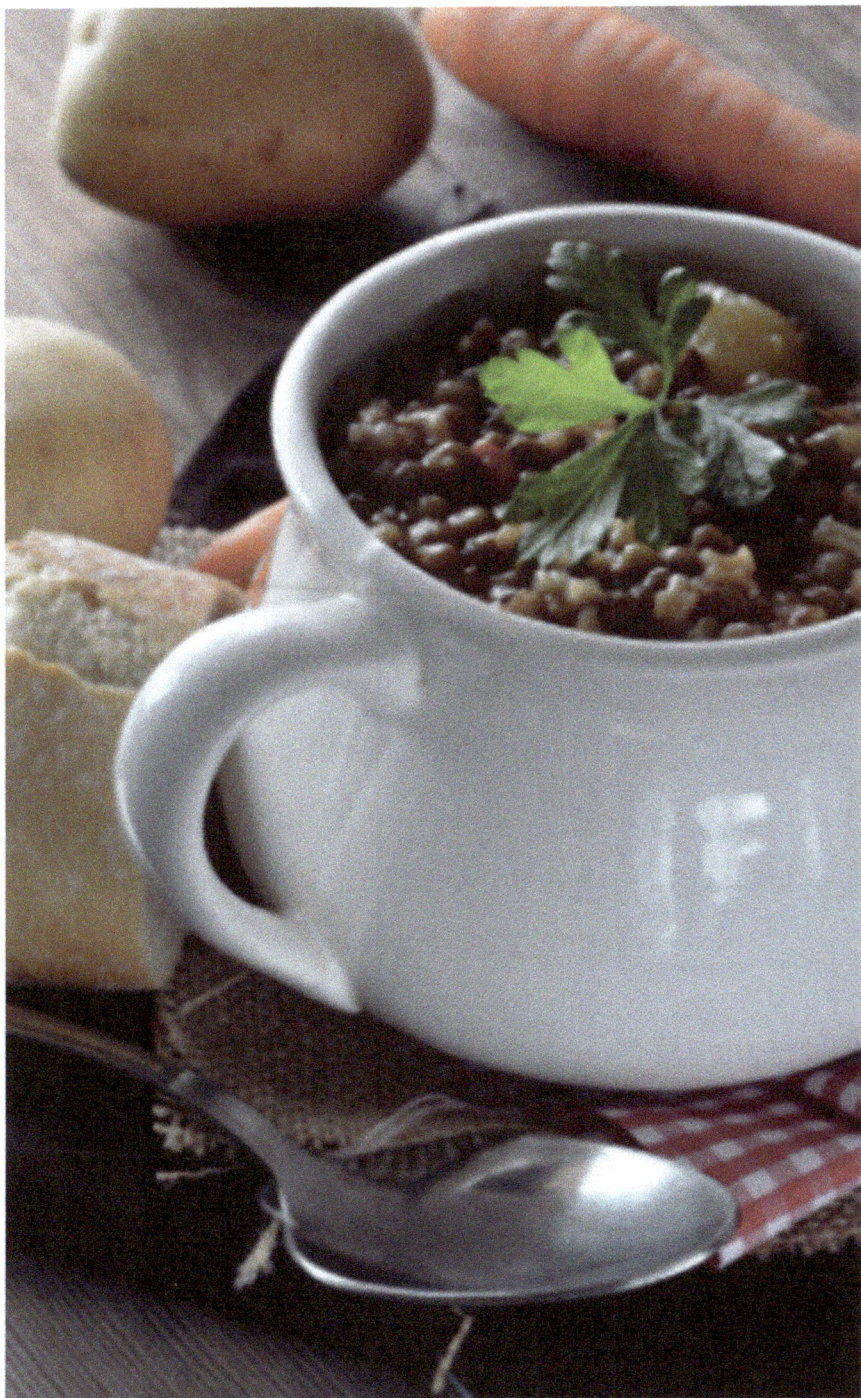

Roasted Garlic and Cauliflower Soup

Preparation Time: 10 minutes

Cooking Time: 35 minutes

Servings: 1-2

Roasted garlic is always a treat, and paired with cauliflower in this wonderful soup, what you get is a deeply satisfy soup with savory, rustic flavors. Blended, the result is a smooth, thick, and creamy soup, but if you prefer a thinner consistency, just adds a little more vegetable broth to thin it out. Cauliflower is anti-inflammatory, high in antioxidants, and a good source of vitamin C (1 cup has 86 percent of your daily value).

Ingredients:

- 4 cups bite-size cauliflower florets
- 5 garlic cloves
- 1½ tablespoons avocado oil
- ¾ teaspoon sea salt

- ½ teaspoon freshly ground black pepper

- 1 cup almond milk

- 1 cup vegetable broth, plus more if desired

-

Directions:

1. Preheat the oven to 450°F. Line a baking sheet with parchment paper.

2. In a medium bowl, toss the cauliflower and garlic with the avocado oil to coat. Season with the salt and pepper, and toss again.

3. Transfer to the prepared baking sheet and roast for 30 minutes. Cool before adding to the blender.

4. In a high-speed blender, blend together the cooled vegetables, almond milk, and vegetable broth until creamy and smooth. Adjust the salt and pepper, if necessary, and add additional vegetable broth if you prefer a thinner consistency.

5. Transfer to a medium saucepan, and lightly warm on medium-low heat for 3 to 5 minutes.

6. Ladle into 1 large or 2 small bowls and enjoy.

__Nutrition:__ Calories: 48; Carbohydrates: 11g; Protein: 1.5g

Beefless "Beef" Stew

Preparation Time: 10 minutes

Cooking Time: 0 minutes

Servings: 4

The potatoes, carrots, aromatics, and herbs in this soup meld so well together, you'll forget there's typically beef in this stew. Hearty and flavorful, this one-pot comfort food is perfect for a fall or winter dinner.

Ingredients:

- 1 tablespoon avocado oil

- 1 cup onion, diced

- 2 garlic cloves, crushed

- 1 teaspoon sea salt

- 1 teaspoon freshly ground black pepper

- 3 cups vegetable broth, plus more if desired

- 2 cups water, plus more if desired

- 3 cups sliced carrot

- 1 large potato, cubed

- 2 celery stalks, diced

- 1 teaspoon dried oregano

- 1 dried bay leaf

Directions:

1. In a medium soup pot over medium heat, heat the avocado oil. Include the onion, garlic, salt, and pepper, and sauté for 2 to 3 minutes, or until the onion is soft.

2. Add the vegetable broth, water, carrot, potato, celery, oregano, and bay leaf, and stir. Get to a boil, decrease the heat to medium-low, and cook for 30 to 45 minutes, or until the potatoes and carrots be soft.

3. Adjust the seasonings, if necessary, and add additional water or vegetable broth, if a soupier consistency is preferred, in half-cup increments.

4. Ladle into 4 soup bowls and enjoy.

Nutrition: Calories: 59; Carbohydrates: 12g

Creamy Mushroom Soup

Preparation Time: 5 minutes

Cooking Time: 20 minutes

Servings: 4

This savory, earthy soup is a must try if you love mushrooms. Shiitake and baby Portobello (cremini) mushrooms are used here, but you can substitute them with your favorite mushroom varieties. Full-fat coconut milk gives it that close-your-eyes-and-savor-it creaminess that pushes the soup into the comfort food realm—perfect for those cold evenings when you need a warm soup to heat up your insides.

Ingredients:

- 1 tablespoon avocado oil
- 1 cup sliced shiitake mushrooms
- 1 cup sliced cremini mushrooms
- 1 cup diced onion

- 1 garlic clove, crushed

- ¾ teaspoon sea salt

- ½ teaspoon freshly ground black pepper

- 1 cup vegetable broth

- 1 (13.5-ounce) can full-fat coconut milk

- ½ teaspoon dried thyme

- 1 tablespoon coconut aminos

Directions:

1. In a great soup pot over average-high hotness, heat the avocado oil. Add the mushrooms, onion, garlic, salt, and pepper, and sauté for 2 to 3 minutes, or until the onion is soft.

2. Add the vegetable broth, coconut milk, thyme, and coconut aminos. Reduce the heat to medium-low, and simmer for about 15 minutes, stirring occasionally.

3. Adjust seasonings, if necessary, ladle into 2 large or 4 small bowls, and enjoy.

Nutrition: Calories: 65; Carbohydrates: 12g; Fat: 2g;
Protein: 2g

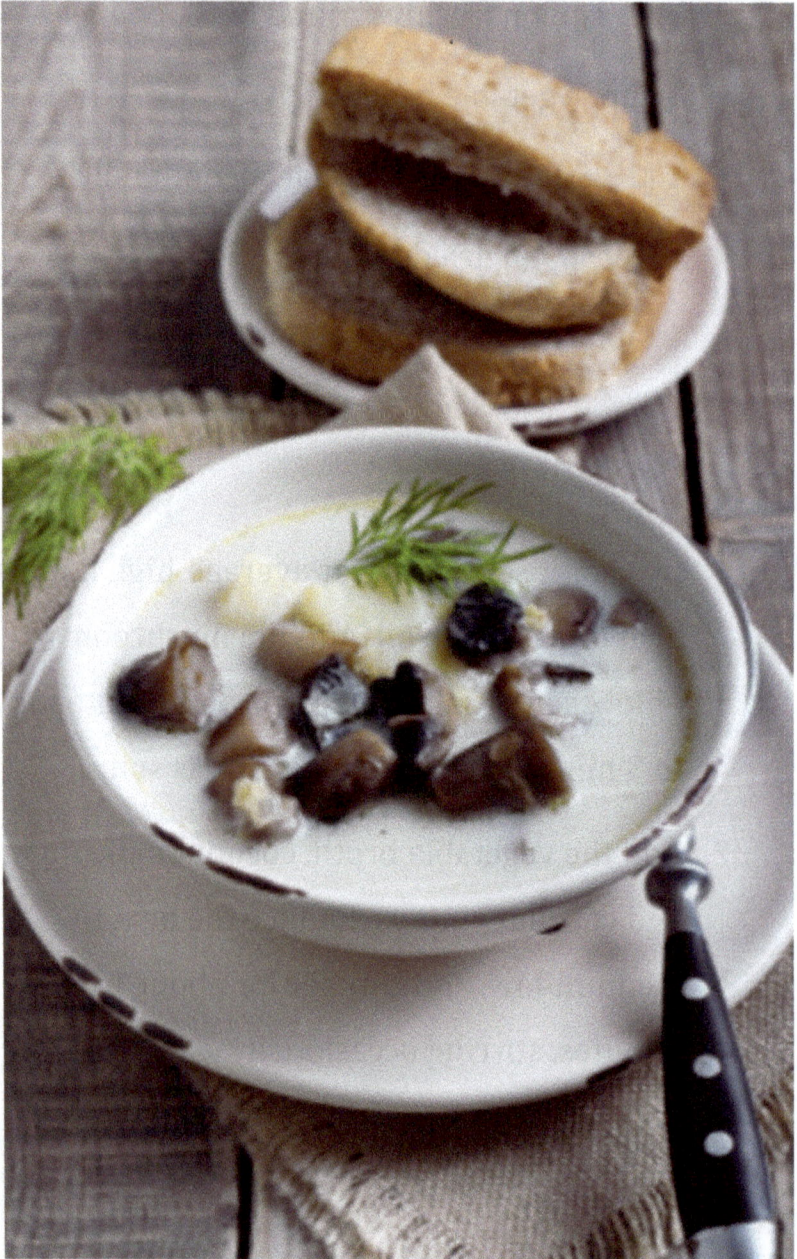

Chilled Berry and Mint Soup

Preparation Time: 5 minutes

Cooking Time: 20 minutes

Servings: 1-2

There's no better way to cool down when it's hot outside than with this chilled, sweet mixed berry soup. It's light and showcases summer's berry bounty: raspberries, blackberries, and blueberries. The fresh mint brightens the soup and keeps the sweetness in check. This soup isn't just for lunch or dinner either—tries it for a quick breakfast, too! If you like a thinner consistency for this, just add a little extra water.

Ingredients:

FOR THE SWEETENER

- ¼ cup unrefined whole cane sugar, such as Sucanat

- ¼ cup water, plus more if desired

- FOR THE SOUP

- 1 cup mixed berries (raspberries, blackberries, blueberries)
- ½ cup water
- 1 teaspoon freshly squeezed lemon juice
- 8 fresh mint leaves

Directions:

1. To prepare the sweetener
2. In a small saucepan over medium-low, heat the sugar and water, stirring continuously for 1 to 2 minutes, until the sugar is dissolved. Cool.

To prepare the soup

3. In a blender, blend together the cooled sugar water with the berries, water, lemon juice, and mint leaves until well combined.
4. Transfer the mixture to the refrigerator and allow chilling completely, about 20 minutes.
5. Ladle into 1 large or 2 small bowls and enjoy.

__Nutrition:__ Calories: 89; Carbohydrates: 12g; Fat: 6g; Protein: 2.2 g

Vegetable Soup

Preparation Time: *10 Minutes*

Cooking Time: 30 Minutes

Servings: *5*

Ingredients:

- 8 cups Vegetable Broth
- 2 tbsp. Olive Oil
- 1 tbsp. Italian Seasoning
- 1 Onion, large & diced
- 2 Bay Leaves, dried
- 2 Bell Pepper, large & diced
- Sea Salt & Black Pepper, as needed
- 4 cloves of Garlic, minced
- 28 oz. Tomatoes, diced
- 1 Cauliflower head, medium & torn into florets
- 2 cups Green Beans, trimmed & chopped

Directions:

1. Heat oil in a Dutch oven over medium heat.

2. Once the oil becomes hot, stir in the onions and pepper.

3. Cook for 10 minutes or until the onion is softened and browned.

4. Spoon in the garlic and sauté for a minute or until fragrant.

5. Add all the remaining Ingredients to it. Mix until everything comes together.

6. Bring the mixture to a boil. Lower the heat and cook for further 20 minutes or until the vegetables have softened.

7. Serve hot.

Nutrition: Calories 79Kl; Fat 2g; Carbohydrates 8g; Protein 2g; Sodium 187mg

Traditional Beef Stroganoff

Preparation Time: 10 minutes

Cooking Time: 30 minutes

Serving: *4*

Ingredients:

- 1 teaspoon extra-virgin olive oil

- 1-pound top sirloin, cut into thin strips

- 1 cup sliced button mushrooms

- ½ sweet onion, finely chopped

- 1 teaspoon minced garlic

- 1 tablespoon whole-wheat flour

- ½ cup low-sodium beef broth

- ¼ cup dry sherry

- ½ cup fat-free sour cream

- 1 tablespoon chopped fresh parsley

Direction:

1. Position the skillet over medium-high heat and add the oil.

2. Sauté the beef until browned, about 10 minutes, then remove the beef with a slotted spoon to a plate and set it aside.

3. Add the mushrooms, onion, and garlic to the skillet and sauté until lightly browned, about 5 minutes.

4. Whisk in the flour and then whisk in the beef broth and sherry.

5. Return the sirloin to the skillet and bring the mixture to a boil.

6. Reduce the heat to low and simmer until the beef is tender, about 10 minutes.

7. Stir in the sour cream and parsley. Season with salt and pepper.

Nutrition: 257 Calories; 6g Carbohydrates; 1g Fiber

Chicken and Roasted Vegetable Wraps

Preparation Time: 10 minutes

Cooking Time: 20 minutes

Serving: *4*

Ingredients:

- ½ small eggplant
- 1 red bell pepper
- 1 medium zucchini
- ½ small red onion, sliced
- 1 tablespoon extra-virgin olive oil
- 2 (8-ounce) cooked chicken breasts, sliced
- 4 whole-wheat tortilla wraps

Directions:

1. Preheat the oven to 400°F.
2. Wrap baking sheet with foil and set it aside.

3. In a large bowl, toss the eggplant, bell pepper, zucchini, and red onion with the olive oil.

4. Transfer the vegetables to the baking sheet and lightly season with salt and pepper.

5. Roast the vegetables until soft and slightly charred, about 20 minutes.

6. Divide the vegetables and chicken into four portions.

7. Wrap 1 tortilla around each portion of chicken and grilled vegetables, and serve.

Nutrition: 483 Calories; 45g Carbohydrates; 3g Fiber

When your body is low on sugars, it will be forced to use a subsequent molecule to burn for energy; in that case, this will be fat. The burning of fat will lead you to lose weight.

www.ingramcontent.com/pod-product-compliance
Lightning Source LLC
Chambersburg PA
CBHW050746030426
42336CB00012B/1689